Sing – sing a song
Sing out loud
Sing out strong
Sing of good things, not bad
Sing of happy not sad
Sing – sing a song
Make it happy
To last your whole life long
Don't care if it's not good enough
For anyone else to hear
Just sing - sing a song

Written by Louis Prima made popular as sung by Karen Carpenter

*Dedicated
to our Family
of Singers*

Sharon and Barry met in Barry's Mom's Church Choir, where they along with Sharon's Mom and Barry's Dad and Sister, followed Mom Towner's (a gold medal contralto in her own right) energetic direction. Growing up singing in church choirs, school choirs and groups, singing was, and continues to be, a big part of their lives. Their love of singing continues through the Sweet Adeline International Society and the Barbershop Harmony Society. Sharon sings with the four time International Gold Medalist North Metro Chorus. Barry sings with the Toronto Northern Lights Chorus, the 2013 Barbershop Harmony Society International Gold Medalists. The love of singing was transferred and encouraged in their home. Questions asked, like what's for dinner? were answered with a song… 'peasandcarrotsmeatloafandpotatoes'…sung to the tune of "Mary had a little lamb"…much to their girls chagrin!

Barry and Sharon's three lovely daughters now also sing and each have four Gold Medals with the North Metro Chorus. Their three wonderful sons-in-law sing in choruses. Their three terrific grandsons sing in the award winning Ontario Youth A cappella (O YA) Chorus founded by Barry and Sharon in 2009. The O YA Chorus encourages young men between the ages of 12 and 30 to sing in a safe, encouraging environment and while doing so enjoy the art form of four part a cappella singing in the Barbershop style. Their three beautiful granddaughters are just waiting their turn to join a chorus.

"the only thing better than singing is more singing"
....Ella Fitzgerald

"he who sings frightens away his ills".....Cervantes

"singing promotes health, breathing, circulation, and digestion".....John Harvey Kellog

We Sing because....

we are happy   we are sad

     we are afraid   we pray

       we celebrate   we learn

    we connect to our souls

we want to heal

    we meditate   we remember

     we want to forget

    we want to pass time

we connect to people   we are creative

     we connect to history

   we politicize   we worship

we feel   we protest

      we share values

we connect to places

    we are human

It's true! Like athletes, not everyone is gifted to be a star... but everyone can and should sing their song. Your stage can be your shower, your car, your kitchen, your garden, your laundry room, work, the local theatre company, the Church Choir, the rock or jazz band, school choir, Glee Club, College Choir, University Choirs and Ensembles, Orpheus Choir, Chamber Choir, Concert Choir, Children's Choir, Barbershop Chorus, your backyard, or Broadway. It is totally OK to just sing!

Human beings are born with the inclination to sing. It is natural and a human birthright.

Barry and Sharon Towner are the founders and principals of
BRING IT ON Performance Coaching
You can contact them at **416 709 3775** or **ssbtowner@aol.com**
www.BringitOnPerformanceCoaching.com

Singing belongs to everyone.
Fill your heart and soul with song.
You'll be glad you did!

SINGING is FUN

Write your own song just by adding a
melody to your thoughts. Make your
melody go up and down, fast and slow,
high and low, any melody you like.
Forget about making sense, how you
sound, or if it's right or wrong. Don't
judge your compositions. Sing your
words and thoughts freely and have
FUN.

'FUN FUN FUN' by Mike Love/Brian Wilson as
performed by the BEACH BOYS

SINGING makes you HAPPY

Singing creates positive energy and a happy mood that is infectious and transparently good for everyone.

'If You're Happy and You Know It Clap Your Hands' by Alfred B. Smith

SINGING is FREE

You can sing anywhere, anytime and it
doesn't cost anything!
You carry your own instrument with
you everywhere you go.
There are no cumbersome cases or parts
to replace!

'Born Free' by John Barry

SINGING boosts SELF ESTEEM

Singing promotes a feeling of achievement. Achievement provides a boost to your self esteem which increases your poise and presentation. Singing helps you feel self assured, in control, physically alive and creative. It feeds your soul as it creates physical well-being. Physical, mental and emotional health is a side effect of singing.

'I will Survive' by Freddie Perren/Dino Fekaris

SINGING tones FACIAL MUSCLES

Singing exercises your facial muscles and keeps you looking younger longer. As you sing you use facial expressions, improving the muscle tone in your face, throat, neck, and jaw. **Warning**: Don't stop singing. Those facial muscles are like any other muscle in your body. When not being used they will wrinkle.

'Baby Face' by Benny Davis/Harry Akst

SINGING encourages
CREATIVITY

Creative singing is freely singing whenever and wherever you are, naturally expressing everything within you. Let emotions flow freely into your voice. Sing and enjoy with your whole being. Do air guitar and sing in the shower. Take your ideas and practice them, and lo and behold, creativity happens. Singing animates the mind, body, and spirit.

'Just Haven't Met You Yet' by Michael Buble / Alan Chang / Amy Foster

SINGING enhances
COMMUNICATION

Singing adds a rich, more pleasant quality to speech and broadens expressive communication. Music is the universal language.

'The Sound of Silence' by Simon & Garfunkel

SINGING improves
CIRCULATION

Singing makes you breathe more deeply
than many forms of strenuous exercise,
carrying more oxygen to your blood
cells, thus improving your circulation.

'Do the Circulation' by Schoolhouse Rock

SINGING exercises the BRAIN

We use different sides of the brain for different activities. Music uses a different side of the brain than language so when you sing you use the two sides of your brain simultaneously to deliver the music and the lyrics.

'If I Only Had a Brain' by Harold Arlen/ E.Y. Harburg from *The Wizard of Oz*

SINGING is AGELESS

Babies are born singing. You can sing throughout your life for free wherever, whenever, and forever. You are never too young or too old to sing! Every human being is, in principle, capable of developing sufficient vocal skills to participate in group singing for a lifetime.

'You Make Me Feel so Young' by Josef Myrow/ Mack Gordon

SINGING tones ABDOMINAL MUSCLES

Singing requires more involvement of the tummy muscles just to sustain a tone than speaking does. The muscles of the back and abdomen aid the diaphragm and lungs in establishing the movements necessary for breathing while you are singing.

'This Little Piggy' English language nursery rhyme

SINGING improves COGNITIVE ABILITY

Singing does make you smarter. Singing enhances the brain's ability to do other things. Learning to sing songs from beginning to end improves reading skills and motor skills. Singing encourages cognitive flexibility and improves mental alertness. Singing stimulates insight into prose and poetry as well as piquing interest in the inner meaning of words. Singing requires focused attention and memorization.

'Twinkle Twinkle Little Star' popular English lullaby

SINGING keeps you YOUNG

Singing keeps you healthier and younger for longer. Singing exercises the vocal cords and keeps them youthful. The less age-battered your voice sounds, the more you will feel and seem younger.

'When you Wish Upon a Star' by Leigh Harline/Ned Washington from *Pinocchio*

SINGING is a PAIN RELIEVER

The endorphins produced help you forget that painful back/knee/tooth or whatever and reduce chronic pain. Singing blocks the neural pathways that the pain travels through.

'Bridge Over Troubled Waters' by Simon & Garfunkel

SINGING means less DOCTOR VISITS

Singing is the best free drug going. It works magic on the brain.

Singing engages many of the body systems (i.e. lungs, heart, nervous system, and brain). It is no surprise that it has such over all benefits.

'Miss Polly had a Dolly' author unknown

SINGING HEALS

Singing is therapeutic emotionally and physically. Singing is helping people dealing with Parkinson's disease, chronic fatigue syndrome, psychiatric disorders, developmental delay, physical disabilities, brain injuries, autism, terminal illness, hearing disorders, auditory or visual impairments, addictions, and abuse issues.

'Somewhere over the Rainbow' by Harold Arlen/ E.Y. Harburg from *The Wizard of Oz*

SINGING is HEALTHY

Singing the **short 'a' sound**, as in <u>AHH</u> for 2-3 minutes will help banish the blues.

To boost alertness, make the **long 'e' sound**, as in <u>E</u>mit.

Singing the **short 'e' sound**, as in <u>E</u>cho stimulates the thyroid gland.

Making the **long 'o' sound**, as in <u>O</u>cean stimulates the pancreas.

Singing the **double 'o' sound**, as in t<u>OO</u> activates the spleen.

'The Sun Will Come Out Tomorrow' by Charles Strouse/Martin Charnin for the musical *ANNIE*

SINGING for your HEART

The singing breath carries more oxygen to your cells, exercises your heart and likely prolongs life due to a lowered heart rate and decreased blood pressure.
There is some evidence that heart rates sync up when singing as a group.

'All You Need is Love' by John Lennon/ Paul McCartney

SINGING boosts IMMUNITY

Singing detoxifies your lymphatic system, thereby supporting your immune system. Singing improves the body's cardiovascular system and reduces the opportunity for bacteria to flourish in the upper respiratory tract, helping to prevent colds and flu.

'I Love to Laugh' by Richard M. Sherman / Robert B. Sherman from *Mary Poppins*

SINGING helps your SINUSES

The exercise of singing opens your sinuses and respiratory tubes. Using your resonators helps to clear the breathing apparatus. Singing clears sinuses and respiratory tubes.

'I'm a Little Teapot' by George Harold Sanders/Clarence Z. Kelley

SINGING is good for your LUNGS

Our lungs never stop working for us. They carry oxygen to the blood and remove toxic gasses 24 hours a day, every day. You do this automatically when you sing out loud whenever and wherever you are. Singing gives your lungs a workout.

'Every Breath You Take' by Sting

SINGING eases RESPIRATORY AILMENTS

Singing encourages asthma and other lung disease sufferers to breathe at a more manageable rate.

'Butterfly Kisses' by Bob Carlisle/Jeff Carson/Raybon Brothers

SINGING improves EYESIGHT

Singing vibrates and aligns the bones of the skull as it massages the eyes and eye muscles. Singing integrates the right and left brain hemispheres which work the visual system for clearer vision.

'The Night has a Thousand Eyes' by Benjamin Weisman/Dorothy Wayne/Marilynn Garrett

SINGING reduces MEDICATION

Singers take fewer medications. The feel good endorphins address issues that might otherwise cause a need for medication.

'Just a Spoonful of Sugar' by Robert B. Sherman and Richard M. Sherman from *Mary Poppins*

SINGING aids SLEEP

Singing acts as a stress reliever. The aerobic exercise derived from singing aids in getting a good sleep. Improving the muscle tone in the larynx helps calm snoring and counters insomnia.

'Brahms' Lullaby' by Johannes Brahms

SINGING is ADDICTIVE

It's not a bad thing! It's good for you. Once you start to sing daily you will miss it if you stop. It's hard to get that feel good feeling anywhere else.

'Sing Sing Sing' written by Louis Prima made famous by Benny Goodman

SINGING is SOOTHING

Parents sing to sick and upset babies. You can sing to calm yourself. Singing calms a terminally ill patient. Researchers are beginning to discover that singing is like an infusion of the perfect tranquilizer, the kind that soothes nerves and elevates spirits.

'These are a few of My Favorite Things' by Rodgers & Hammerstein from *The Sound of Music*

SINGING promotes
CONFIDENCE

Regardless of what you sound like, love your voice. Be open and accepting of your own voice. It's the only one you'll ever have. Sing from your heart. You have a right to sing and the world needs you to sing.

'The Grand Old Duke of York' English children's nursery rhyme

SINGING improves MEMORY

Singing strengthens your concentration skills and memory. Learning new songs, or memorizing the words to familiar songs boosts the level of acelylcholine associated with memory and strengthens the brain.

'Memories' by Andrew Lloyd Webber

SINGING is POWERFUL

Singing is risk free, economic, easily accessible and a powerful road to enhanced physiological and psychological well-being.

'Climb Every Mountain' by Rogers and Hammerstein from *The Sound of Music*

SINGING reduces DEPRESSION

Singing is the best anti-depressant on the market. Depression, anger and anxiety is reduced when singing, if not completely released.

Singing boosts the release of endorphins and oxytocin which help relieve depression.

"Music has charms to soothe a savage breast."

Seventeenth century poet William Congreve

'Whistle a Happy Tune' by Rogers and Hammerstein for the musical *The King and I*

SINGING improves POSTURE

Your posture will improve as you sing. Your chest expands and your back and shoulders straighten as you break into song. Be the puppet, feel the string from the top of your head down your spine.

'Got No Strings' by Leigh Harline/Ned Washington from Disney's *Pinocchio*

SINGING expresses EMOTION

Singing provides a catharsis across the full emotional spectrum. Music, "the universal language", stirs our deepest emotions. A level of freedom is reached emotionally when singing. Think about it. For every situation there is a line from or a title of a song that you probably already know.

'Get Happy' by Harold Arlen/Ted Koehler

SINGING improves ENERGY

Singing out loud requires an intake of breath. Sing a full song and there's plenty of extra oxygen pumping into your system to help you feel energized. Singers generally see an increase in their other activities and see life with an added zest.

'42nd Street' by Al Dubin/Harry Warren for the musical by the same name

SINGING is ENRICHING

Singing enriches your ability to appreciate the art of great singers. Singing enriches your imagination. Singing encourages sensitivity and understanding. Singing helps maintain your well-being and happiness. Singing stretches you out of your comfort zone and daily routine.

Singing is, therefore, fundamentally enriching.

'Singing in the Rain' by Al Dubin/Harry Warren for the musical by the same name

SINGING is EASY

Your body houses your vocal
instrument.
Just start by humming then sing your
words and thoughts...like....
'hmmmmmIthinkI'lldolaundrytoday '.
It is just sustained speech...easy!

'Easy Street' by Alan Rankin Jones/Carlton

SINGING is in FASHION

Thanks to the popularity of hit shows such as "Glee", "American Idol", "America's got Talent", "Canada's got Talent", "Britain has Talent", "The Voice" and others of that genre, singing is now a cool thing to do.

'You're never Fully Dressed without a Smile'
by Charles Strouse/ Martin Charnin from *Annie*

SINGING shares HISTORY

Before there were governments or nations, tribes and groups used song and dance to build loyalty to the group, transmit vital information and ward off enemies. Those who sang well survived. Before written language emerged, critical stories were passed on in song. The Hebrew Torah, the Greek Myths, the Iliad, and the Odyssey were all sung before they were ever written down. When we sing we tap into something that is one of the most ancient of human practices.

'Circle of Life' by Elton John/Tim Rice from Disney's film *The Lion King*

SINGING enhances LEARNING

Preschool and kindergarten teachers have known for a long time that children learn best through songs. They remember the material and message better and it is easier to keep them engaged in the activity. Singing improves your ability to 'listen'.

'Alphabet Song' author unknown

SINGING is MEDITATION

Singing helps you 'let go'. When you surrender to the voice within, you transcend your physical self, just as in other forms of meditation. The effects of singing are at a deeply unconscious level which on a normal day to day activity level is impossible to reach.

'Dream a Little Dream of Me' by Milton Adolphus/Wilbur Schwandt/Fabian Andre/ Gus Kahn

SINGING releases STRESS

Singing takes your mind off the stresses of the day, and yes, those endorphins that are released in the brain act as mood lifters. The full singers breath (diaphragmatic) used while singing aids in relaxation of body and mind and releases muscle tension.

'Shaking the Blues Away' by Irving Berlin

SINGING connects us to PLACES

It may be a birth place, ancestral location, favorite place or city. Did you leave your heart in San Francisco or give your regards to Broadway?

'I left My Heart in San Francisco' by George Cory/Douglas Cross
'New York New York' by John Kander/Fred Ebb
'Bali Hai' by Rodgers and Hammerstein for the musical *South Pacific*

SINGING to PROTEST

Protest songs are frequently situational or may be abstract, expressing opposition to injustice and support for peace or free thought. In all cases they express a human passion, a capacity for feeling pain and pleasure, and hence empathy.

'If I had a Hammer' by Pete Seeger/Lee Hays

SINGING shares VALUES

Singing unites factions, religions and races. Group singing is cheaper than therapy, healthier than drinking and more fun than working out! You may go to rehearsal exhausted and depressed, but by the end of the rehearsal you walk out high on endorphins and good will.

'True Colors' by Billy Steinberg/Tom Kelly

SINGING PRAISES

Worship by song is an ancient tradition in all cultures. One of the best ways we can express being filled with the "Spirit" (joy) is by singing psalms, hymns, spiritual songs and national anthems.

'Oh When the Saints Go Marching In' American gospel hymn origin unknown

SINGING brings JOY

Experience the joy of producing and being part of a beautiful sound. Singing from the heart and the pure delight of your own voice and song brings joy! Sing for the joy of living.

'Joy to the World' by Isaac Watts/Lowell Mason adapted in 1839 from an older melody which was then believed to have originated from Handel

SINGING is SOCIAL

Join a group, community or church choir and widen your circle of friends. Sharing the joy of singing will enrich your life far beyond the notes and music.

From the histories of very ancient cultures, singing, eating and dancing has been a crucial activity in the bonding of groups of people and in teaching, customs, worship, partying and socializing.

'Auld Lang Syne' by Robert Burns and set to the tune of a traditional folk song

SINGING engages the WHOLE BODY

It takes your whole body to support your voice. You need to use your core muscles to support the production of your sound.

'Do the Hokey Pokey' children's action song

SINGING builds COMMUNITY

Join a community or church choir. The world will never turn down a song, especially when it comes from the heart.

'With A Song in My Heart' by Rodgers and Hart

SINGING CELEBRATES

We celebrate Christmas, Hanukkah, Valentine's Day, St. Patrick's Day, Easter, National Holidays, Birthdays, and other holidays with songs that are passed down traditionally from generation to generation in our worldwide variety of cultures. From early childhood we associate songs with family, warm gatherings, special food, smells and special times.

'Happy Birthday to You'   the most recognized song in the English language

SING Just **BECAUSE**

You can!!!!!